Primordial Strength Systems Basic Middle Age Explosive Power Endurance

By Steven Helmicki

To Dr. Mohan Ramanchandran, Dr. Tibby Hunt, and Dr. Jenny Garafalo:
Your hard work and continuous feedback has led to another Primordial chapter.
Your progress and improvement has been beyond any expectations.

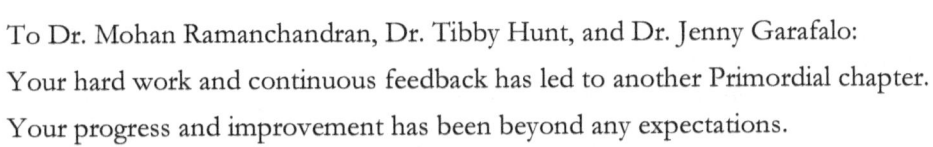

Male trainees add 10% more resistance and volume.

Record all workouts in the Primordial Training Log.

Phase M54- two workouts

Work-Out #1

Prehab with 5lb pullovers x 10 bent x 10 straight and mini-band internal/external shoulder rotation (25reps each arm)

Leg raises- 10reps

Glut/ham/calf raise-5reps

Rapid succession 6sets: 1 bodyweight jump Immediately Followed By 2 squats with 4kg

Mini-band stiff-legged deadlift-10reps

Band Good Mornings mini-band-10-reps

Shrugs-4kgs-3sets of 5reps with 3sec rest b/w sets

Stiff leg dead lifts-4kgs-2sets of 6reps with 3sec rest b/w sets

Bicep curls-5lbs-3sets of 5reps (all 3 hand positions) palms up, hammer, reverse

Band face pulls (light band)-3sets of 5reps with 3sec rest b/w sets

Band Chest pulls (mini- band)-3sets of 5reps with 3sec rest b/w sets

Medicine Ball neck (forward/back)-6reps each

Sit-ups-15 reps-5lb medicine ball

Repeat again during the week.

Phase M 55

Work-Out

Prehab

Bodyweight Box squats-3sets of 5reps w/5sec rest

4kg stiff leg dead lifts-3sets of 5 w/3sec rest

Mini-Band Good Morning-10 reps

Kettlebell Bent rows 2reps x 4kg/1 rep x 8kg repeat 4 times

Kettlebell Military Press-2reps x 4kg immediately followed by 1 rep with 6kg repeat 4 times

Band Face pulls-10 reps

Chest pulls-10 reps

Bent arm lateral raises 2lbs-15 reps

Front arm raises 2lbs-15 reps

Shoulder push backs 2lbs-15 reps

Shrugs 4kg-5, 2, 2, 5, 4 w/3sec rest

Bench press 4kg-4sets of 5 reps w/3sec rest

Hammer curls 10lbs-6sets of 2resp w/3sec rest

Curls 10lbs-5, 3, 2, 1, 1, 1, 4 w/4sec rest

Iron cross curls 2lbs-5, 4, 2, 1, 1, 4 w/3sec rest

Mini-band curls-10 reps

Push-downs – 4 sets of 3 reps mini/2 reps monster mini/1rep light IFB 20 reps mini-band

Triceps kickbacks 2lbs-5, 2, 1, 1, 1, 4 w/3sec rest

Triceps extensions 4kgs-5sets of 3reps w/3sec rest

2kg curl/triceps extension-3sets of 5reps no rest

3kg curl/tricepa extension-2sets of 3reps

Swings-3sets of 3 reps 1kg/2 reps 2kg/1rep 4kg

Sit-ups-3 reps BW/3 reps 1kg/5 reps 2kg/5 reps 1kg/ 4 reps 3kg/2 reps 5kg

Standing Abs (purple band)-3 sets of 5 reps straight and to each side

Figure 8s 4kg-12 reps

Repeat twice more during the week

Phase M 56

Work-Out

Knee tracking 2", 10"

Prehab

10" box-5 sets x2 jumps IFB 2 squats

17" box 4kg squats-5, 3, 2, 2, 2, 2, 3, 6 w/3sec rest

Stiff leg dead lifts 4kg-3, 2, 2, 2, 1, 1, 5 w/3sec rest

Bent rows-4sets of 2 reps 4kg/ 1 rep 8kg

Bent rows 4kg-5, 3, 3, 2, 2, 5 w/3sec rest

Curls 4kg-6, 3, 2, 2, 2, 3, 2, 4 w/3sec rest

Reverse curls (mini- band)-10, 4, 3, 2, 2, 2, 10 w/3 sec rest

Iron cross curls 2lbs-6, 3, 3, 2, 2, 6 w/3sec rest

Hammer curls 2lbs-10, 3, 3, 3, 2, 6 w/3sec rest

Shoulder press 6kg-5, 2, 2, 2, 3, 2, 5 w/3sec rest

Face pulls (monster mini- band)-5, 2, 3, 2, 2, 4 w/3sec rest

8kg 4 sets of 3 shrugs/2 high pulls

Bench:

       2lbs straight arm-10, 3, 3, 5, 2, 2, 2, 10 w/3sec rest

       2lbs bent arm pull-over-6, 3, 3, 3, 3, 6 w/3sec rest

       2lbs straight arm pull-over-10 reps

Triceps push-downs-4sets of 3 mini- band/2 reps monster mini-band

Mini- band push-downs-6, 2, 2, 4, 2, 2, 6 w/3 sec rest

4kg Triceps extension-6sets of 2reps w/5sec rest

2lbs Triceps extension 20 reps

Standing abs-4 sets 5 reps mini- band/3 reps monster mini- band

Swings-3sets of #2 4kgs/#1 6kgs

4kg swings-3, 2, 2, 1, 1, 2, 6 w/3sec rest

3 sets of 8kg 5 side bends (each side)/5 figure 8s

Medicine ball smashes-3sets of 3 3kg/1 6kg IFB 12 reps with 2kgs

Punching bag-jab/straight right combo 20 IFB 2/1 10 w/jog

repeat twice more per week.

Phase M 57

Work-Out

Prehab

10" box-4 sets of 1 BW jump IFB 2 reps 4kg squat IFB 1 rep 8kg squat

Stiff leg dead lifts-4 sets of 2 4kg/1 8kg

Bent rows 4kg-5 sets of 5reps w/5sec rest

Swings-6sets of 2 reps 4kg/1 rep 8kg

Chins-2, 1, 1 w/10sec rest

Mini band rows-5sets 2 reps each arm

Face pulls (mini band)-10, 2, 2, 2, 2, 4, 2, 2, 6 w/ 3sec rest

Overhead press 4kg-5, 2, 2, 2, 2, 5 w/3sec rest

2lbs front raises, lateral raises, shoulder push backs-2sets of 5reps each

High pulls 4kgs-5, 2, 2, 2, 1, 1, 3 w/3sec rest

Shrugs- 5 reps 4kg/5 reps 8kg IFB 3 reps 4kg/3 reps 8kg

Curls-4sets of 2 reps 2lbs/ 1 rep 4kg IFB 2lbs 15 reps

Mini-Band curls (to head)-10, 2, 2, 2, 2, 6, 2, 2, 10 3 seconds rest

Bench-4kg 15 reps IFB bent arm pull overs 12 reps

Triceps push downs-4sets of 3 reps mini-band, 2 reps, monster mini, 1 rep light

Triceps extensions-4sets of 2 reps 2kg ball/1 rep 4kg ball IFB 1kg 15 reps

Triceps kickbacks 2lbs-10, 2, 2, 2, 10 w/3sec rest

Bar leg-ups-10 reps each leg IFB 8 reps w/2kg ball

Standing abs-15 reps straight and to each side

Swings-4sets of 3 reps 2kg/2 reps 4kg/1 rep 8kg

Sit-ups-20 rep BW IFB 6sets of 1 rep 2kg ball w/3sec rest IFB 6 reps 2kg ball

Progressive smashes-5 reps 2kg/5 reps 3kg/5 reps 4kg

Side bends 4kg-10 reps each side

Figure 8s-8 reps 4kg/5 reps 6kg/3 reps 8kg

Swings 1kg-20 reps

Repeat twice more per week

Phase M 58

Work-out

Stiff leg dead lifts-4sets of 2 reps 4kg/2 reps 6kg/ 2 reps 8kg

10" box squats-6sets of 2 reps BW/2 reps 4kg

Bent rows-6sets of 2 reps 4kg/2 reps 6kg

Chin/Pull up-alternate 1 rep w/5sec rest

Overhead press-4sets of 2 reps 4kg/2 reps 6kg

High pulls 4kgs-2, 4, 1, 2, 4 w/3sec rest

Front raises 21/2lbs-8sets of 2 reps w/3sec rest

Lateral raises 21/2lbs-6sets of 2 reps w/3sec rest

Push backs 21/2lbs-6sets of 2 reps w/3sec rest

Lateral fly 21/2lbs-4sets of 2reps w/3sec rest

Shrugs 8kgs-5, 3, 2, 1, 5 w/3sec rest

Face pulls (red band)-12reps

Curls 4kgs-4sets of 2 reps 4kg/1 rep 6kg IFB 5sets of 2 reps 2kg ball/2 reps 4kg ball

Iron cross curls /2lbs-12 reps

mini band curls-12 reps

Tricep extensions-3sets of 2 reps 4kg/1 rep 6kg IFB 4kgs 3, 2, 1, 1, 1, 4 w/3sec rest

Push downs-4 sets of 4 reps mini- band/2 reps monster mini- band IFB 5sets of 3 reps mini- band w/3sec rest

Swings-3sets of 2 reps 4kg/2 reps 6kg/2 reps 8kg

Standing abs (light band)-5 reps straight and each side IFB 2, 1, 2 w/3sec rest straight and each side

Smashes 4kgs-3sets of 5 reps w/5sec rest

Figure 8s 8kgs-8 reps

Side bends 8kg x 12 reps each side

Upright rows (mini-band)-15 reps

Light Band Good Mornings-10, 3, 2, 1, 4 w/3sec rest

16" box squats BW-20 reps

Repeat twice more per week

Phase M 59

Work-Out

Stiff leg dead lifts 8kg-#8 IFB 3, 3, 2, 2, 1, 1, 6 w/4sec rest

12" box squats-3 BW IFB 4sets of #2 4kg/#1 6kg IFB #15 BW

Swings 1kg-3, 2, 3, 1, 1, 6 w/3sec rest

Step-ups 12" box-#5 4kg/#5 6kg each leg

Overhead press-4sets of #2 4kg/#1 6kg IFB 4kg 3, 2, 1, 1, 3, 1, 4 w/3sec rest

High pulls-4sets of #2 4kg/#1 6kg

Shrugs-8sets of #4 4kg/#2 6kg/#18kg

Bent rows-4sets of #4 purple band/#4 6kg

Curls-4sets of #2 4kg/#1 6kg IFB 4kgs 2, 1, 2, 1, 3, 1, 1, 4 w/3sec rest IFB 21/2lbs #15

Black band curls (standing under foot)-#10

Being held face curls-#10

Triceps extension-4sets of #2 4kgs/#1 6kgs IFB 4kgs 3, 2, 1, 1, 3, 1, 1, 6

Face pulls-3, 5, 2, 2, 7 w/3sec rest

Swings-4sets of #2 4kg/#1 6kg IFB 4kg 3, 2, 1, 1, 3, 1, 6 w/3sec rest

Side bends 8kg-#8 each side IFB #8 figure 8s

Swings-4sets of #3 1kg/#2 2kg/#1 3kg IFB 1kg 3, 5, 2, 1, 6

Smashes-3sets of #3 1kg/#2 2kg/#1 3kg

Wall throws 2kg-3, 2, 1, 1, 1, 5 w/3sec rest

Black band pull through-#10

Calf raises 8kgs-5, 3, 3, 2, 2, 4, 2, 7 w/3sec rest

Black band overhead tricep extension-#10

Bent laterals 21/2lbs-3, 3, 2, 1, 5 w/3sec rest

Curl/Tricep extension combo 2kg-#5 each IFB #8 each IFB #10 each

Repeat two more times per week.

Phase M 60

Work-Out

Prehab

10" box jump #1 IFB 12" box squat 6kgs-5sets

Stiff leg dead lift-5sets of #2 4kg/#2 6kg/#2 8kg

Bent rows-4sets of #3 4kg/ #3 6kg/#3 8kg

Overhead press-3sets of #2 4kg/#2 6kg/#2 8kg

Dead lift to high pull-3sets of #1 4kg/#1 6kg/#1 8kg

Shrugs-4sets of #2 4kg/#2 6kg/#2 8kg/#2 12kg

Chins-5sets of #1 w/5sec rest

Curls-5sets of #2 4kg/#2 6kg IFB 4kgs 3, 1, 3, 1, 1, 3, 1, 6 w/3sec rest

Triceps extension-4sets of #2 4kg/#2 6kg IFB 4kg 4, 1, 4, 1, 4, 1, 6 w/3sec rest

Push downs black band-5, 2, 5, 2, 5, 2, 6 w/3sec rest

High face pulls black band-#15

Swings-5sets of #2 4kg/#2 6kg/#2 8kg

Smashes 4kg ball-#10

Smashes 2kg ball-#15

Side bends-4sets of #2 4kg/#2 6kg/#2 8kg each side

Figure 8s-#10 12kgs/#12 8kgs/#15 4kgs

Repeat two more times per week.

Phase M 61-repeat two weeks.

Work-Out

Prehab

12" box-5sets of #2 BW squats IFB #2 4kgs IFB #15 BW box squats

Stiff leg dead lifts-5 sets of #2 4kg/#2 6kg/#2 8kg

Bent rows-4sets of #1 4kg/#1 6kg/#1 8kg

Pullovers-#5 straight arm/#5 bent arm

Chins-6sets of #1 w/5sec rest

Dead lift to high pulls-3sets of #1 4kg/#1 6kg/#1 8kg

Curls-4sets of #4 red band curls/#4 4kg

Curls 21/2lbs-#15

Iron cross curls 21/2lbs-#15

Reverse curls 21/2lbs-#15

Overhead press-4sets of #2 4kg/#2 6kg

Shrugs-5reps of #2 4kg/#2 6kg

Push downs red band-#15 long IFB short push downs 5, 2, 5 2, 5 w/3sec rest

Tricep extension 4kgs-#10 IFB 3, 3, 1, 1, 3, 5, 10 w/3sec rest

Face pulls red band-#10 IFB 5, 2, 5, 2, 10 w/3sec rest

Bench 4kgs-#10 overhead/#10 perpendicular/#10 reverse

Tricep extension 21/2lbs-#15

Push-ups-#10 on half ball

Smashes 3kgs-#15

Swings 4kg-#10 IFB 2, 2, 2, 2, 2, 10 w/3sec rest

Bar leg lifts-5 each side, 2 each side, 8 each side w/3sec rest

Three times per week training.

Phase M 62-repeat two weeks.

Work-out #9

Dead Lifts	4kg, 6, 8kg 2 each, 4 sets
Squats 10"	2xBW, 2x4kgs, 6sets
Bent Rows	4kgsx2, 6kgsx2, 6sets
2 Chins/2 Pulls	5sec rest in between
Overhead Press	2x4kg, 2x6kg, 4sets
High P-ulls	4kgs – 2, 4, 1, 2, 4 3sec rest
21/2lbs	Front raises #2 x 8, 3sec rest
	Lateral raises #2 x 6, 3sec rest
	Pushbacks #2 x 6, 3sec rest
	Lateral fly #2 x 4, 3sec rest
Shrugs	8kgs 5, 3, 2, 1, 5, 3sec rest
Face Pulls	Red band #12
Curls	4kgsx2, 6kgsx1, 4sets
	Ball 2kgx2, 4kgx2, 5 sets w/3sec rest in between
21/2lbs Iron X	#12
Curls	Red band #12
Tricep Extension	4kgx2, 6kgx1, 3sets
	4kgs – 3, 2, 1, 1, 1, 4, 3sec rest
Tricep Pushdowns	#4 red, #2 black, 4sets
	Red #3, 5sets with 3sec rest in between
Swings	4kgs#2, 6kgs#2, 8kgs#2, 3sest
Standing Abs	Purple #5 – straight and to each side, then 2, 1, 2 w/3sec rest straight & to each side
Smashes	4kg ball x 5, 3 sets w/5sec rest
Figure 8's	8kgs x 8
Sidebends	8kgs x 8 each side
Leg Band Upright Rows	Red #15
Band Good Mornings	10, 3, 2, 1, 4, 3sec rest
Squats	16" x 20

Three times per week training.
Phase M 63-repeat two weeks.

Work-out

Squats	2xBW, 2x6kg, 4sets
Dead Lifts	4kgx2, 6kgx2, 12kgx2, 3sets
Bent Rows	4kgx4, 6kgx4, 4sets
Landmine Press	45lbs straight up #5 each arm, then 1 each arm x 3 w/gusto
High Pulls	1x4kg, 1x6kg, 3sets
Shrugs	3x4kg, 3x6kg, 3x12, 3sets
Face pulls	Black band #15
Curls	2x4kg, 2x6kg, 4sets
	21/2lbs #20
Reverse Curls	Black band #15
Hammer Curls	21/2lbs #15
Tricep Extensions	4kgs – 6, 2, 2, 2, 4
Tricep Pushdowns	Black band 10, 2, 1, 1, 2, 1, 5
Swings	2x4kg, 2x8kg, 3 sets
Figure 8's	8kg #10 each leg
Landmine Twist	#10 each side
Standing Abs	Black/Purple – 5 each, 3 sets
Smashes	2kgs, #20
Leg-ups	#5 each side, then #10 both legs

Train three times per week.

Phase M 64- repeat two weeks.

Work-out

Prehab

Pullovers

Knee Tracking

Dead lifts	2x4kg, 2x6kg, 2x8kg, 3sets
Bar Squats	#3, 4 sets w/15sec rest, then #1, 3sest with 5sec rest
Trampoline	#1, 3 sets w/5sec rest
Bent Rows	3x4kg, 3x6kg, 3sets
High Pulls	1x4kg, 1x6kg, 2sets
Shrugs	5x4kg, 5x6kg, 5x8kg, 3sets
Face Pulls	Black band – 3, 3, 3, 5 w/5sec rest
Overhead Press	4kg – 2, 2, 2, 2, 2, 6 w/3sec rest
Curls	4kgs – 2xbicep, 2xhammer, 2xreverse, 2sets
	Black band - #15 bicep, #15 reverse
Tricep Extension	2x4kg, 1x6kg, 3sets
Tricep Pushdowns	Green band – 5, 1, 1, 1, 1, 4 w/3sec rest
	Red band - #20
Swings	2x4kg, 2x6kg, 3sets
Side Bends	2x4kg, 2x6kg, 2x8kg, 2sets

Train three times per week.

Phase M 65-repeat two weeks.

Work-out #12

Prehab	
Sumo Squats	2x4kg, 2x8kg, 2x16kg, 3sets
Vertical Jumps	1xBW, 1x4kg, 3sets
Stiff Leg Dead Lifts	2x6kg, 2x12kgs, 3sets
Nautilus Pullover	40lbs #8
Lat Pull Downs	60lbs #8
Shrugs	3x4kg, 3x8kg, 3sets
Overhead Press	2x4kgs, 5sets w/4sec rest
Face Pulls	Black band – 3, 1, 3, 1, 3 w/3sec rest
Curls	Bicep - 1x4kg, 1x6kg, 4sets
	21/2lbs Hammer #20
Tricep Pushdowns	Black/Purple – 2 each, 4 sets, then black band #15
Shrugs	1x4kg, 1x6kg, 1x8kg, 3sets
Figure 8's	8kgs #8
Smashes	2kg #10
Standing Abs	Green band - #5 each position, 2sets
Side Bends	4x4kg, 4x8kg, 3sets
Leg Ups	#5 each leg (alternate) and then 5 both legs

Train twice weekly.

Phase M 66-repeat two weeks.

Work-out #13

Sumo Dead Lifts	2x4kg, 2x6kg, 2x8kg, 3sets
	1x6kg, 1x8kg, 1x12kg, 2sets
Bent Rows	3x6kg, 3x8kg, 2sets
Supinated Pulldowns	40lbs #12
Nautilus Pullovers	30lbs #12
Shrugs	4x8kg, 4x12kg, 2sets
Overhead Press	4kgs – 2, 2, 2, 2, 2 w/3sec rest
Face Pulls	Black band #20
Curls	2x4kg, 2x6kg, 2sets
	4kgs #10
	Black band #10
	Reverse curls black band #10
Tricep Pushdowns	Black band - #10, 2, 2, 2, 2, 10 w/3sec rest
	Purple band - #10, 1, 1, 4 w/3sec rest
Swings	1x4kg, 1x8kg, 4sets
Side Bends	2x4kg, 2x8kg, 2sets
Standing Abs	Purple band - #10 each position
Figure 8's	8kg #10 per leg
Smashes	1kg ball #10
Leg-ups	#8 each leg then #8 both legs

Train twice weekly.

S   W   O   T

S   W   O   T

S   W   O   T

S   W   O   T

S W O T

S   W   O   T

S   W   O   T

S   W   O   T

S   W   O   T

S   W   O   T

S   W   O   T

S W O T

S   W   O   T

S   W   O   T

S   W   O   T

S   W   O   T

S   W   O   T

www.ingramcontent.com/pod-product-compliance
Lightning Source LLC
Chambersburg PA
CBHW031335290526
45784CB00014B/2756